# YOUR KNOWLEDGE HAS VALUE

AF139826

- We will publish your bachelor's and master's thesis, essays and papers

- Your own eBook and book - sold worldwide in all relevant shops

- Earn money with each sale

Upload your text at www.GRIN.com and publish for free

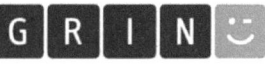

**Bibliographic information published by the German National Library:**

The German National Library lists this publication in the National Bibliography; detailed bibliographic data are available on the Internet at http://dnb.dnb.de .

**Imprint:**

Copyright © 2018 GRIN Verlag
Print and binding: Books on Demand GmbH, Norderstedt Germany
ISBN: 9783668789487

**This book at GRIN:**

https://www.grin.com/document/439127

Ervelio Olazabal

# Intelligent Analysis of Cellular Pathologies in the Blood as a Diagnostic method of Diseases

GRIN Verlag

**GRIN - Your knowledge has value**

Since its foundation in 1998, GRIN has specialized in publishing academic texts by students, college teachers and other academics as e-book and printed book. The website www.grin.com is an ideal platform for presenting term papers, final papers, scientific essays, dissertations and specialist books.

**Visit us on the internet:**

http://www.grin.com/

http://www.facebook.com/grincom

http://www.twitter.com/grin_com

**Ervelio E Olazabal,**

# "Intelligent" Analysis of Cellular Pathologies in the Blood as a Diagnostic Method of Diseases

# TITLE: "Intelligent" Analysis of Cellular Pathologies in the Blood as a Diagnostic Method of Diseases.

"WEXXON MEDICAL RESEARCH". Miami, Fl, USA.

## SUMMARY:

The current methodologies and diagnostic procedures make it possible to detect diseases, pathological states, assess risk, evolution, severity, complications incidences, recovery of the patient and possible toxic damage caused by drug candidates, and other therapeutic products, because it is feasible to compare normal cells with patterns of these in their pathological state in peripheral blood, skin and other tissues and organs. These results are achieved by manual and automated methods that manage to detect a large number of diseases, and anomalous states, even when they have disadvantages, and "errors", which restrict the diagnosis of some diseases that directly affect the health of patients and drug research processes. These techniques are based on the analysis of the variations of the forms, quantities, inclusions and transitions of colors, among other peculiarities that differentiate normal cells from sick or damaged cells. In search of more effective and efficient diagnostic solutions, mathematical algorithms have been developed that enable the processing of "Visual" images and "Pattern Recognition" to apply the "Automatic Learning" techniques that allow the "Intelligent" recognition of the differences between stereotyped and anomalous cells with the help of computational tools that in turn allow to increase the speed of the analysis without losing sensibility, as well as to diminish the cost of the same one.


**KEYWORDS:** Blood smear, diagnosis, hematomorphology, diseases, hematological software.

# Inhalt

# 1. INTRODUCTION.

The analysis of normal cells present in peripheral blood, skin and other organs and tissues, in humans and animals, and the consequent comparison of these with patterns of the same lineages, in their pathological state, allow to diagnose numerous diseases and at the same measure to evaluate the risk, evolution, severity, complications incidence and recovery of the patient (1,2,3,4,5,6,7).

This is possible because the variations in the forms, values, inclusions, and transitions of colors, among other cellular peculiarities that in the singular and combinations become pathological patterns, are the result of the transformations, and variations, of the metabolic and anomalous processes in tissues and organs that can be interpreted, and visually correlated, with the help of the microscope by hematologists, histologists and pathologists to provide indispensable information so that doctors apply protocols aimed at prevention, treatment, cure and remission of acute, chronic diseases and to reverse the process of organ and tissue aging (8,9,10).

These same attributes, of the cells, are used by automated machines to count, detect and compare most of the differences that occur between cells, normal and pathological, with an enough high accuracy level which allow that the specialists might guide to issue confident medical diagnoses. It must be noted that these methods will never achieve what a trained human eye can achieve (8,11).

The combination of visual and automated procedures, although both have their limitations (12,13,14), have become invaluable tools to assist physicians and related personnel in making decisions about the application of the best procedures and protocols to follow, in each patient in a personalized way, for the prevention and treatment of diseases, as well as to elucidate the toxic effects that drug candidates might cause, and other therapeutic products of commercial interest, during the process of their research and development (15,16,17,18,19,20,21,22).

However, despite the fact that the achievements that have been obtained with the application of these methods of analysis are unquestionable, at present not all social sectors have "full" access to the diagnosis of the diseases that cause the greatest incidence and morbidity; due to the limited number of specialists trained to execute visual exams, the costs of the studies and the recurring "errors" that are usually implicit in the automated equipment currently used for such purposes, as well as the inability of these to detect a significant number of diseases. The aforementioned results in the impossibility of carrying out massive surveys of communities and populations, which ultimately limits the process of early detection, prevention and treatment of diseases; and to the same extent, the research and development of new patent medicines and other therapeutic products by the institutions dedicated to this activity are affected.

The restrictions implicit in the diagnostic, visual and automated methods, which reduce the diagnostic effectiveness and the number of drugs and products to be evaluated, were taken into consideration by our team of scientists and professionals, dedicated to the development of patent medicines (23, 24,25,26,27,28,29,30), to develop and compose an "intelligent" computer tool that eliminates the insufficiencies that the diagnostic, visual and automated processes show, and meets all the expectations and needs that doctors and researchers require for the diagnosis of diseases and pathological states respectively.

The procedure was based on the development of mathematical algorithms, and image processing, which have the ability to compare normal cells with patterns of those same strains in a pathological state. The matching process is based on the qualities, quantities, morphology and polychromaticism among other features that the "intelligent" tool uses to significantly reduce the "errors" that make the diagnostic technologies used up to the present, still show deficiencies in the diagnoses (31,32,33).

## 2. BACKGROUND OF THE UTILITY OF PERIPHERAL BLOOD SMEAR FOR THE DIAGNOSIS OF DISEASES.

The microscopic examination of an appropriately prepared and well-reviewed blood smear by a professional expert in the laboratory is necessary and clinically useful in a variety of circumstances and for a variety of reasons. In this article, we attempt to delineate the purpose and criteria for the examination of blood smears in a variety of circumstances found in the daily practice of the hematology laboratories. A blood smear test is used at least to: (a) verify the marked automatic hematology results and (b) determine if a manual differential count of leukocytes is necessary. The blood smear / manual differential white blood cell (CBC) examination provides the complete haematological assessment of the case, at least from the morphological point of view.

Reviewing the blood smear with or without interpretation serves to ensure that no clinically significant findings are omitted, in addition to providing a diagnosis or a diagnostic clue, particularly if interpreted by a physician (34). In order to arrive at the diagnosis of the diseases it is necessary to first determine the morphological alterations that the formed elements of the blood present (Leukocytes, Red Blood Cells and Platelets) that are summarized in Table No.1.

**Table No.1. Main morphological alterations of red blood cells (35, 36,37)**

**Red blood cells.**

| Morphological alteracions | Number | Morphological alteracions | Number | Morphological alteracions | Number |
|---|---|---|---|---|---|
| **Blood Red cells** | | | | | |
| Anocytosis | > 3+ | Eliptocytes | > 3+ | Rouleaux | > 2+ |
| Poikilocytosis | > 3+ | Stomatocytes | > 3+ | Tear cells | > 1+ |
| Hypochromia | > 3+ | Microcytes | > 2+ | Schistocytes | > 1+ |

| Polychromasia | > 3+ | Macrocytes | > 2+ | Spherocytes | > 1+ |
|---|---|---|---|---|---|
| Basophilic stippling | > 3+ | Target cells | > 2+ | Acanthocytes | > 1+ |

Sickle cells, Howell Jolly bodies, Pappenheimer bodies and agglutinations.

## White blood cells

| Dohle bodies | > 3+ | Hiposegmented neutrophils | > 2+ | Hypersegmented neutrophils | > 1+ |
|---|---|---|---|---|---|

Hypogranular granulocytes,
Auer rods

Toxic granules,
Left shift

## Platelets

| Giant platelets | > 2+ | Platelet satelitosis | | | |
|---|---|---|---|---|---|
| | | Thrombocytopenia, Thrombocytosis | | | |

## Other cells or organisms

| Basophilic (%) | > 4+ | Atypical lymphocytes (%) | > 10+ | Blasts (%) | > 10+? |
|---|---|---|---|---|---|
| Promyelocytes (%) | > 3+ | Myelocytes (%) | > 5+ | Metamyelocytes (%) | > 10+ |
| Other abnormal cells or any non-identifiable, nucleated red blood cells | > 2+ | Organisms | Any | | |

The group of diseases that it can be diagnosed presumptively it is quite extensive and includes the following groups of diseases (Table No.2).

**Table No.2. Diseases that are can be diagnosed by a blood smear manually reviewed under the optical microscope (38, 39, 40, 41, 42).**

| Benign diseases | Malignant diseases |
|---|---|
| Hereditary and acquired anemias. | Acute leukemias. Hematological disorders secondary to hepatopathies and chronic illness. |
| Immunological and secondary thrombocytopenia. | Chronic leukaemias. |
| | Biphenotypic and bilineal leukemia, |
| Bacterial, viral, fungal infections and parasites. | Medullary insufficiency syndrome. |
| Congenital and acquired neutropenia. | Chronic myeloproliferative Disorders. |
| Autoimmune diseases. | Primary hypereosinophilias. |
| | Paroxysmal nocturnal hemoglobinuria. |
| | Discretion of plasma cells. |

## 3. TRANSCENDENCE OF THE METHODS OF PERIPHERAL BLOOD DIAGNOSTICS.

The results emanating from laboratory analyzes are feasible for their purposes when the referrals are correct, reliable, effective, efficient and relevant without impairing quality for the diagnosis and monitoring of patients, and also for epidemiological studies, surveillance of public health and for the development and research of new medicines and other products (1,6,11). Up to now, the analysis of a peripheral blood sample can be carried out using visual methods, with the help of a microscope, and using automated equipment that is capable of counting a very high number of cells per unit of time (40,43).

Although automated analyzers promote fairly accurate results for all hematological parameters, to the point that they have drastically decreased the use of visual blood smear methods; these have disadvantages and diagnostic limitations related to the underdiagnoses or overdiagnoses of diseases or pathological states because they are not able to differentiate in details the stage of development or maturity in which certain cell lines are found; obviate elements or morphological changes that when viewed are considered pathological; they do not detect inclusions in the red and white blood cells; they are susceptible to interferences associated with metabolic states or medication of patients; they interpret the instantaneous changes of some formal elements as pathological and "report" false positive results, which definitely make them register as atypical cells or "alarm" all those parameters that are impossible to process (1, 33).

In this sense, the well trained human eye remains irreplaceable at present. It does not mean that manual differential counting is not subject to errors that, although in a lesser extent, also affect the results and effectiveness of the diagnosis (1,34), mainly those related to the fatigue of the specialist.

Precisely, for these reasons, recently an international consensus has been reached to harmonize criteria, on validation standards, which will result in significant savings in response time and cost, as well as material and human resources when conducting peripheral blood studies for diagnose diseases. Within accepted diagnostic processes, we find those that presuppose the processing of images, blood smear, through the use of computer tools that use advanced algorithms to achieve these purposes (1).

## 4. ASPECTS THAT LIMIT THE METHODS OF PERIPHERAL BLOOD DIAGNOSTICS

Most clinical laboratories worldwide have drastically decreased and / or eliminated the peripheral blood diagnosis from the visualization of a smear of this tissue. This place has been occupied by automated self-analyzers that have advantages and limitations in relation to manual processing (12, 14).

Among the disadvantages, presented by automated equipment, is the fact that they do not detect poikilocytosis or erythrocyte inclusions; they are susceptible to interferences that alter the results due to Lipemia, Severe Jaundice, Hemolysis, Auto agglutination by Cold Antibodies and Leukemias, among others; report false positive results related to platelet alterations because they change shape from the moment of their extraction, as well as the presence of giant platelets among other alterations of this series that definitely suggest the need for any platelet alteration should be analyzed again in manual form because automated counting can be altered by pseudotrombocitopenias, microcytes, erythrocyte fragments, intraerythrocytic inclusions, microcoagula, heparin, among others; Interferences in the automatic counts of the white series due to the presence of cryoglobulins, cryofibrinogen, monoclonal proteins, erythroblasts, platelet aggregates, unlysed erythrocytes, micro clots and circulating heparin, among others (34,35,36). By On the other hand, manual (visual) counting using the microscope also has its drawbacks as a result of errors in the preparation and staining of the smear, in cell distribution, in cellular interpretation and in the number of cells counted (37,38).

## 5. RATIONALE FOR "SMART" TOOLS FOR THE PROCESSING OF IMAGES

The disadvantages of manual and automated methods, for the analysis of peripheral elements in peripheral blood, are presented as an opportunity to look for solutions that help correct these deficiencies, at the same time that we can take the positive attributes, and the advantages, that these procedures present to develop more efficient "smart" tools. In the specific case of shape  elements, present in peripheral blood, it is

9

feasible to develop algorithms depending on the number, composition, different types and subtypes, shapes and different tones that in the singular or combinations are feasible to detect, and compare, through and with the help of digital microscopes that enable "Visual" processing and "Pattern Recognition"; considered indispensable elements to apply the techniques of "Automatic Learning" that allow the "Intelligent" recognition of the cells by assistance of computational tools (45,46,47).

In general, the process of automated observation, of shape elements, includes the acquisition of peripheral blood samples, visualization of these using digital microscopes, location of the cells, segmentation of the area of these, extraction of characteristics, classification and analysis. Several studies have addressed the task of locating blood-forming elements as the first step in this process. In this sense, the best results are achieved through the use of simple methods that in a unique way or compositions are based on the threshold techniques of Global Theshold, Otsu Thresholding (48), Region Growing (49), Watershed (50). Methodologies established and subject to the distribution of the intensity of the pixels in the image.

The certainty of these methods depends on the contrast between the object and its background. Threshold methods are widely used, since there is a high contrast between the nucleus of the cells in relation to the background. However, it must be borne in mind that in the case of other objects in the image with intensities similar to cells or elements formed for analysis objects, then we might have  wrong results by the presence of false positives.

The classification also applies " Haar Cascade "which is a technique developed by Viola Jones (51,52). This is based on "haar-like" features that is combined with an accelerated cascade classifier. The peculiarity "haar-like" is widely used for the detection of objects, which provides a rapid extraction process and capable of processing low resolution images. This method has been satisfactorily applied in several object detection tasks, including the detection of style (53, 54, 55).

In this review we can not fail to mention one of the methods that has been most approached in achieving the objectives that they pursue. "intelligent" programs for the diagnosis of peripheral blood smears We refer to the "Software" called "CellaVision Peripheral Blood Application" that has the ability to extract images from digital cells and delivers a pre-classification / pre-characterization of these lineages using innovative technology of Artificial Neural Network, which have the ability to visualize the classes of cells side by side, or all cells in a full screen view, adjusts the magnification of the images of the cell, compare the cells with images of reference cell of a built-in reference library, label or add comments to any slide, type of cell or specific cell; it exports and sends by email cell images for consultation, validation or presentation; when re-sorting is needed, then the cells are easily dragged and placed in the appropriate cell category and archive cell images as part of the patient's image and medical history. All of which accelerates the process of review and verification by a medical technologist and consequently the diagnosis of diseases (56).

The aforementioned procedures and techniques served as the basis for our team of researchers to develop a method to detect shape elements in peripheral blood samples, through a software solution capable of handling large volumes of data in a short time and capable of overcoming, Through Deep Learning techniques, human efficiency in this type of tasks.

## 6. LIMITATIONS OF CURRENT INTELLIGENT TOOLS AND NEW APPLICATIONS FOR THE DIAGNOSIS IN PERIPHERAL BLOOD FROTIS.

It was recognized by the group of experts in hematology of ICSH that manual diagnosis is more precise and less subjective than the diagnoses made by machines (57).

Overcoming this conflict introduces a paradigm that must be overcome and currently constitutes a challenge for researchers, who work in this area, and also justifies working hard to solve this problem, based on blood smear analysis, due to the advantages offered by it (58). For example, after the storage time is set, it can be more or less long, compared with other blood preservation methods, maintaining the morphological integrity of the cells that make up the blood (59). Based on the above, our objective of work, taking into account the limitations and advances of the laboratory equipment used up to the present, is to create a simple and automated system of high performance for the classification of morphology and other peculiarities of blood cells.

This system is already in its final phases of development, evaluation and validation. Currently we use it as a computer tool to help hematopathologists, who work in our team, but soon we will put it on the market as a high performance and effective tool for the hematological diagnosis. This software is capable of diagnosing morphological alterations with precision in red blood cells, all types of leukocytes, and platelets, as well as recognizing the parasitosis present in a blood smear. The digital processing is carried out from the introduction of the images of each smear in the software with a processing level above 60 images per minute. A report of 4 pages of each patient is also automatically issued,  where the most likely diagnosis, the alterations found and the complementary diagnosis suggestions and 4 pictures of the smears evaluated with the alterations found.

These results are reviewed by a hematopathologist before being delivered as a diagnosis. No doubt the advances made to the present in the intelligent diagnosis of blood smear images, have served to validate currently a software that allows to accelerate the process of haematological diagnosis, starting from the blood smear as a primary sample, decreasing costs and the response time, increasing the sensitivity and specificity of the same. Everything that we will publish in another article dedicated specifically to the software that we are concluding.

# 7. CONCLUSIONS

Diagnostic processes are supported by the analysis of normal cells and the consequent comparison with patterns of the same lineages in their pathological state in the skin, peripheral blood, tissues and organs. The diagnostic methods used, at present, for the analysis of cells present in peripheral blood show limitations and errors that limit the diagnoses of several diseases. It is feasible to develop mathematical algorithms for the processing of "Visual" images and "Pattern Recognition", and then apply the techniques of "Automatic Learning" that consent "Intelligent" recognition of cells with the help of computational tools. The development of intelligent tools for diagnostic imaging has allowed us to approach the launch of software that will be very useful for hematopathologists, which we will do in another publication.

# 8. REFERENCES.

1. Hoffman R, Benz EJ, Silberstein LE, Heslop K, Weitz J, Anastasi J. Haematology. Basic Principles and Practice Approach. Philadelphia, PA: Elsevier. Seventh edition. 2018.

2.    Greer JP, Arber DA, Glader B, List AF, Means RJ, Parashevas F, Rodgers GM. Examination of the Blood and Bone Marrow. In: Wintrobe's Clinical Hematology. 13th. ed. Philadelphia: Lippincott Williams & Wilkins; 2014. p. 9-35.

3.    Tarek Elghetany M, Banki KM. Erythrocytic disorders. In: McPherson RA, Pincus MR. Henry's Clinical Diagnosis and Management by Laboratory Methods. Philadelphia: Elsevier Saunders; 2011. p. 557-99.

4.    Means R: Anemias Secondary to Chronic Diseases and Systemic Disorders. In: Greer JP,Arber DA, Glader B, et al. Wintrobe's Clinical Hematology. Philadelphia: Lippincott Williams & Wilkins; 2013. p. 2307-41.

5.    Ham R, Sloane D, Warshaw GA, Potter JF, Flaherty E. Anemia. In: Ham´s Primary CareGeriatrics. Philadelphia: Elsevier Saunders; 2014. p. 491-6.

6.    Choccalingam, C., R.K.N. Radha, and N. Snigdha, Estimation of Platelet Counts and Other Hematological Parameters in Pseudothrombocytopenia Using Alternative Anticoagulant: Magnesium Sulfate. Clin Med Insights Blood Disord, 2017. 10: p. 1179545X17705380. https://www.ncbi.nlm.nih.gov/pmc/articles/PMC5428203/.

7.    Choi AH, Bolaris M, Nguyen DK, Panosyan EH, Lasky JL, Duane GB. Clinicocytopathologic correlation in an atypical presentation of lymphadenopathy with review of literature. Am J Clin Pathol. 2015;143(5):749-54.

https://academic.oup.com/ajcp/article/143/5/749/1761971.

8.    Vives Corrons JL, Aguilar I, Bascompte JL. Examen morfológico de las células sanguíneas. In: Vives Corrons JL, Aguilar I, Bascompte JL. Manual de técnicas de laboratorio en hematología. 4ta. ed. Barcelona: Masson; 2014. p. 59-104. 5.

9.    Courville EL, Crisman S, Linden MA, Yohe S. Green Neutrophilic Inclusions are Frequently Associated With Liver Injury and May Portend Short-Term Mortality in Critically Ill Patients. Lab Med. 2017:48(1):18-23.

https://www.ncbi.nlm.nih.gov/pubmed/?term=Green+Neutrophilic+Inclusions+are+Fre
quently+Associated+With+Liver+Injury+and+May+Portend+Short-
Term+Mortality+in+Critically+Ill+Patients.

10.    Dayton VJ, et al. Relapsed Acute Promyelocytic Leukemia Lacks "Classic" Leukemic Promyelocyte Morphology and Can Create Diagnostic Challenges. Am J Clin Pathol. 2017;147(1):69-76.
https://www.ncbi.nlm.nih.gov/pubmed/28108472.

11.    Newman AW, Rishniw M, Behling-Kelly E. Reporting and interpreting red blood cell morphology: is there discordance between clinical pathologists and clinicians? Vet Clin Pathol. 2014:43(4):487-95.
https://www.ncbi.nlm.nih.gov/pubmed/25280365.

12.    Pierre RV. Peripheral blood film review: The demise of the eyecount leukocyte differential. Clinics in Laboratory Medicine. 2002;22(1):279–97.
https://www.ncbi.nlm.nih.gov/pubmed/11933579.

13.    Borzova E, Dahinden CA. The absolute basophil count.    Methods Mol Biol. 2014;1192:87-100.
https://www.ncbi.nlm.nih.gov/pubmed/25149486.

14.    Briggs C, Culp N, Davis B, d'Onofrio G, Zini G, Machin SJ. ICSH guidelines for the evaluation of blood cell analysers including those used for differential leucocyte and reticulocyte counting. Int J Lab Hematol. 2014;36(6):613-27.
https://www.ncbi.nlm.nih.gov/pubmed/24666725.

15.    Cortés R, Morales A, Reiner T, Aguila E. Estudio de hemosiderina en bazos de diferentes especies animales para la investigación científica. Revista. Medicentro. 1995;12(2).
16.    Cortés R, Perez JA, et al. Some toxicological issues of the ophtalmic oinment QUERATOFURAL. Journal of Veterinary pharmacology and therapeutic. Vol.20,1997.
http://agris.fao.org/agris-search/search.do?recordID=GB1997029681.

17.     Cortés R, Pérez J, Olazabal E. ¿Biofuncionalales versus envejecimiento de la piel. ¿son correctas las estrategias actuales? Revista Cubana de Farmacia. 2008;42(3).

18.     Dueñas A, Cortés R, Marrero O, Pérez J A, Olazabal E. Toxicidad aguda del extracto hidroalcohólico de la planta Chuquiragua Jussieui Administrado por vía oral en ratas.          Revista          La          Técnica.          2013:(10):12-17. https://revistas.utm.edu.ec/index.php/latecnica/article/view/559.

19.     Dueñas A, Alcibar U, Olazabal E, Cortés R.  Efecto antioxidante de la Chuquiraga jussieui J. F. Gmel en el ensayo de hemólisis. Revista Medicentro.2014;18(2). http://www.medigraphic.com/cgi-bin/new/resumenI.cgi?IDARTICULO=48459.

20.     Dueñas A, Alcibar U, Olazabal E, Cortés R. Análisis Fitoquímico y de Seguridad de los Extractos de Chuquiraga Jussieui JF. Gmel, Revista Centro Agrícola. 2014;41(2).http://cagricola.uclv.edu.cu/index.php/es/volumen-41-2014/numero-2-2014/32-analisis-fitoquimico-y-de-seguridad-de-los-extractos-de-chuquiraga-jussieui-j-f-gmell.

21.     Montero-Torres A, García-Sánchez RN, Marrero-Ponce Y, Machado-Tugores Y, Nogal-Ruiz JJ, Martínez-Fernández AR,  Arán VJ, Ochoa C,  Meneses-Marcel A, Torrens F. Non-stochastic quadratic fingerprints and LDA-based QSAR models in hit and lead generation through virtual screening: theoretical and experimental assessment of a promising method for the discovery of new antimalarial compounds. Send toEur J Med Chem.                                        2006;41(4):483-93.https://www.sciencedirect.com/science/article/pii/S0223523406000353?via%3Dihub.

22.     Marrero-Ponce Y, Meneses-Marcel A, Castillo-Garit JA, Machado Y, Escario JA, Gómez-Barrio A, Montero D, Nogal JJ, Arán VJ, Martínez-Fernández AR, Torrens F, Rotondo R, Ibarra-Velarde F, Alvarado YJ. Predicting antitrichomonal activity: A computational screening using atom-based bilinear indices and experimental proofs. Bioorg.          Med.          Chem.          2006;14(19):6502–6524. https://www.sciencedirect.com/science/article/pii/S0968089606004718?via%3Dihub.

23.     Meneses-Marcel A, Rivera-Borroto OM, Marrero-Ponce Y, Alina Montero A, Machado Tugores Y, Escario JA, Gómez A, Montero D, Nogal JJ, Kouznetsov VV, Ochoa C, Bohórquez AR, Grau R, Torrens F, Ibarra-Velarde F, Rotondo R, Alvarado IJ, Vogel C,

Rodriguez-Machin L. New Antitrichomonal Drug-like Chemicals Selected by Bond (Edge)-Based TOMOCOMD-CARDD Descriptors. J Biomol Screen. 2008;13(8): 785-794. http://journals.sagepub.com/doi/abs/10.1177/1087057108323122?url_ver=Z39.88-2003&rfr_id=ori%3Arid%3Acrossref.org&rfr_dat=cr_pub%3Dpubmed&

24.     Marrero-Ponce Y, Cabrera-Pérez MA, Romero-Zaldivar V, Bermejo-Sanz M, Siverio-Mota D, Torrens-Romero F. Prediction of Intestinal Epithelial Transport of Drug in (Caco-2) Cell Culture from Molecular Structure using 'in silico' Approaches During Early Drug Discovery. Internet Electronic J Mol Des. 2005;4:124-150. http://www.biochempress.com/av04_0124.html.

25.     Medina-Marrero R, Castillo-Garit JA, Romero-Zaldivar V, Torrens F, Castro EA. Protein Linear Indices of the "Macromolecular Pseudograph's α-Carbon Atom Adjacency Matrix" in Bioinformatics. Part 1. Prediction of Protein Stability Effects of a Complete Set of Alanine Substitutions in Arc Repressor. Bioorg. Med. Chem. 2005, 13, 3003-3015. http://www.mdpi.com/1420-3049/9/12/1124.

26.     Torrens F, Martínez Y, Romero-Zaldivar V, Castro EA. Atom, Atom-type, and Total Non-Stochastic and Stochastic Quadratic Fingerprints: A promising approach for modeling of antibacterial activity. Bioorg Med Chem. 2005;13(8):2881-2899. https://www.sciencedirect.com/science/article/pii/S096808960500129X?via%3Dihub.

27.     Castillo-Garit JA, Nodarse D. Linear Indices of the Macromolecular Graph's Nucleotides Adjacency Matrix as a Promising Approach for Bioinformatics Studies. 1. Prediction of Paromomycin's Affinity Constant with HIV-1 Ψ-RNA Packaging Region. Bioorg Med Chem. 2005;13(10):3397-3404.https://www.sciencedirect.com/science/article/pii/S0968089605002051?via%3Dihub.

28.     González-Díaz H, Olazabal E, Santana L, Uriarte E, González-Díaz Y, Castanedo N. QSAR study of anticoccidial activity for diverse chemical compounds: prediction and experimental assay of trans-2-(2-nitrovinyl) furan. Bioorganic & medicinal chemistry. 2007;15(2):                                                      962-968. https://www.sciencedirect.com/science/article/pii/S0968089606008662.

29.	Marrero-Ponce Y, Castillo-Garit JA, Olazabal E, Serrano H, Morales A, Castanedo N, Ibarra-Velarde F, Huesca-Guillen A, Sánchez AM, Torrens F, Castro EA. Atom, atom-type and total molecular linear indices as a promising approach for bioorganic and medicinal chemistry: theoretical and experimental assessment of a novel method for virtual screening and rational design of new lead anthelmintic. Bioorganic & medicinal chemistry. 2005;13(2): 1005-1020. https://www.sciencedirect.com/science/article/pii/S0968089604009411.

30.	González Díaz H, Olazabal E, Castañedo N, Hernádez I, Morales A, Serrano H, González J, Ramos de Armas R. Markovian chemicals "in silico" design (MARCH-INSIDE), a promising approach for computer aided molecular design II: experimental and theoretical assessment of a novel method for virtual screening of fasciolicides. Molecular modeling.2002;8(8):237–245.	https://link.springer.com/article/10.1007/s00894-002-0088-7.

31.	Da Rin G, Vidali M, Balboni F, Benegiamo A, Borin M, Ciardelli ML, Dima F, Di Fabio A, Fanelli A, Fiorini F, Francione S, Germagnoli L, Gioia M, Lari T, Lorubbio M, Marini A, Papa A, Seghezzi M, SolarinoL, Pipitone S, Tilocca E, Buoro S. Performance evaluation of the automated nucleated red blood cell count of five commercial hematological analyzers. International Journal of Laboratory Hematology. 2017;39(6):663-670. Wiley Online Library

32.	S. Pipitone L, Germagnoli G, Da Rin A, Di Fabio A, Fanelli F, Fiorini S, Francione A, Marini A, Papa A, Benegiamo T, Lari F, Siviero M, Lorubbio M, Borin M, Seghezzi ML, Ciardelli F, Dima M, Buoro S. Comparing the performance of three panels rules of blood smear review criteria on an Italian multicenter evaluation, International Journal of Laboratory Hematology. 2017;39(6):645-652. Wiley Online Library

33.	Chari PS, Prasad S. Study on the Performance of a New System for Image Based Analysis of Peripheral Blood Smears on Normal Samples. Indian J Hematol Blood Transfus.2018:34(1):125-131. https://www.ncbi.nlm.nih.gov/pubmed/?term=Study+on+the+Performance+of+a+New+System+for+Image+Based+Analysis+of+Peripheral+Blood+Smears+on+Normal+Samples#.

34.    Gulati G, Song J, Florea AD, Gong J. Purpose and criteria for blood smear scan, blood smear examination, and blood smear review. Ann Lab Med. 2013;33(1):1-7. https://www.ncbi.nlm.nih.gov/pmc/articles/PMC3535191/.

35.    Retamales CE. Recomendación para la interpretación del frotis sanguíneo del subprograma de morfología sanguínea. Santiago de Chile: Instituto de Salud Pública. Laboratorio Nacional de Referencia de Hematología; 2013.1-20. Disponible en: http://www.ispch.cl/sites/default/files/interpretacion frotis sanguineo - 14052013A.pdf.

36.    Constantino BT. Reporting and grading of abnormal red blood cell morphology. Int    J    LabHem.    2014;    37    (1):    1-9.    Disponible    en: http://onlinelibrary.wiley.com/doi/10.1111/ijlh.12215/pdf.

37.    Gulati GL, Alomari M, Kochar W, Schwarting R. Critera for blood smear review. Lab    Med    2002;33:374-7.    Disponible    en: https://academic.oup.com/labmed/article/33/5/374/2657226.

38.    Alteraciones en el extendido de sangre periférica. Revista de Inmunoalergia 2014;12 (2):1-9. Disponible en:

39.    Gulati G. Blood Cell Morphology Grading Guide, 3rd edn. Chicago, IL: American Society for Clinical Pathology Press. 2009:1–45. http://freeofread.com/download/blood-cell-morphology-grading-guide/

40.    Palmer L, Briggs C, Mcfadden S, Zinis G, Icsh J, Burthem G, Ozenberg M, Proytcheva M, Machine SJ. Recommendations for the standardization of nomenclature and grading of peripheral blood cell morphological features. Int Jnl Lab Hem. 2015;37:287–303. http://www.qualitat.cc/sitebuildercontent/sitebuilderfiles/2015-IJLH.pdf.

41.    Bull BS, Herrmann PC. Morphology of the erythron. In: Hematology, 4th edn. Kaushansky K, Beutler E, Seligsohn U, Lichtman MA, Kipps TJ, Prchal JT (eds). New York: McGraw Hill; 2010: 409–27.

42.    Glassy EF. Color Atlas of Hematology An Illustrated Field Guide Based on Proficiency Testing. CAP Hematology and Clinical Microscopy Resource Committee. Northfield,IL: College of American Pathologists.1998.

43.    Cornet, E., et al., Evaluation and optimization of the extended information process unit (E-IPU) validation module integrating the sysmex flag systems and the recommendations of the French-speaking cellular hematology group (GFHC). Scand J Clin                Lab                Invest.                2016;76(6):465-71. https://www.ncbi.nlm.nih.gov/pubmed/?term=Evaluation+and+optimization+of+the+e xtended+information+process+unit+(E-

IPU)+validation+module+integrating+the+sysmex+flag+systems+and+the+recommen dations+of+the+French-speaking+cellular+hematology+group.

44.    Loddo A, Di Ruberto C, Kocher M. Recent Advances of Malaria Parasites Detection Systems Based on Mathematical Morphology. Sensors (Basel). 2018;18(2): pii: E513. doi: 10.3390/s18020513.

http://www.mdpi.com/1424-8220/18/2/513.

45.    Riedl JA, Stouten K, Ceelie H, Boonstra J, Levin MD, van Gelder W. Interlaboratory Reproducibility of Blood Morphology Using the Digital Microscope. J Lab Autom.                2015;20(6):670-5. htttp://journals.sagepub.com/doi/abs/10.1177/2211068215584278?url_ver=Z39.88- 2003&rfr_id=ori%3Arid%3Acrossref.org&rfr_dat=cr_pub%3Dpubmed&

46.    Constantino BT. Reporting and grading of abnormal red blood cell morphology. Int J LabHem [revista en Internet]. 2014 [ cited 6 May 2016 ] ; 37 (1): [aprox. 9p]. http://onlinelibrary.wiley.com/doi/10.1111/ijlh.12215/pdf.

47.    Nazlibilek S, Karacor D, Ercan T, Sazli MH, Kalender O, Ege Y. Automatic Segmentation, Counting, and Classification of White Blood Cells. Measurement. 2014;55:58-65.

https://www.researchgate.net/publication/262018755_Automatic_Segmentation_Counti ng_Size_Determination_and_Classification_of_White_Blood_Cells.

48.    Nemane JB, V.A. Chakkarwar VA, P.B. Lahoti PB. White Blood Cell Segmentation and Counting using Global Theshold. International Journal of Emerging Trends & Technology in Computer Science (IJETTCS). 2013;3(6):639-643.

http://citeseerx.ist.psu.edu/viewdoc/download?doi=10.1.1.413.2998&rep=rep1&type=p df.

49.    Duan J, Yu L. A WBC Segmentation Method Based on HIS Color Space. Proc. 4 th IEEE International Conference on Broadband Network and Multimedia Technology (IC-BNMT). 2011:629-632.

50.    Chourasiya S, Rani GU. Automatic Red Blood Cell Counting Using Watershed Segmentation. International Journal of Computer Science and Information Technologies (IJCSIT). 2014;5(4):4834-4838.

https://pdfs.semanticscholar.org/ef24/ae99ca56cdb65d66d23cf3767ee8a73972d7.pdf

51.    Viola P, Jones M. Rapid object detection using a boosted cascade of simple features. Proceeding of Conference on Computer Vision and Pattern Recognition. 2001;1:511-518.

http://wearables.cc.gatech.edu/paper_of_week/viola01rapid.pdf

52.    Viola P, Jones M, Snow D. Detecting pedestrians using patterns of motion and appearance. Int J Comput. 2005:63(2):153–161.

https://dl.acm.org/citation.cfm?id=1057318.

53.    Yeong K, Hwang SY. An improved Haar-like feature for efficient object detection. Pattern Recognition Letters. 2014;42:148-153.

https://www.sciencedirect.com/science/article/pii/S0167865514000658.

54.    Landesa-Vázquez, J Alba-Castro. The role of polarity in Haar-like features for face detection. Proceedings of International Conference on Pattern Recognition. 2010;412–415.

https://ieeexplore.ieee.org/document/5597819/.

55.    Li Y, Lu W, Wang S, Ding X. Local Haar-like features in edge maps for pedestrian detection. Proceedings of International Congress Image and Signal Processing. 2015;3:1424–1427.

https://ieeexplore.ieee.org/document/6100477/

56.    Cellavision Home Page. 2018. https://www.cellavision.com/en/

57. Comar SR, Malvezzi M, Pasquini R. Evaluation of criteria of manual blood smear review following automated complete blood counts in a large university hospital, Revista Brasileira de Hematologia e Hemoterapia. 2017;39(4):306-317. Crossref

58. Terry NR, Mendoza CA. Importancia del estudio del frotis de sangre periférica en ancianos. Medisur 2017;15(3):20p. http://www.medisur.sld.cu/index.php/medisur/article/view/3597.

59. Cutts T, Cook B. Poliquin G, Strong J, Theriault S. Inactivating Zaire Ebolavirus in Whole-Blood Thin Smears Used for Malaria Diagnosis. J Clin Microbiol. 2016.54(4):1157-9. http://jcm.asm.org/content/54/4/1157.long.

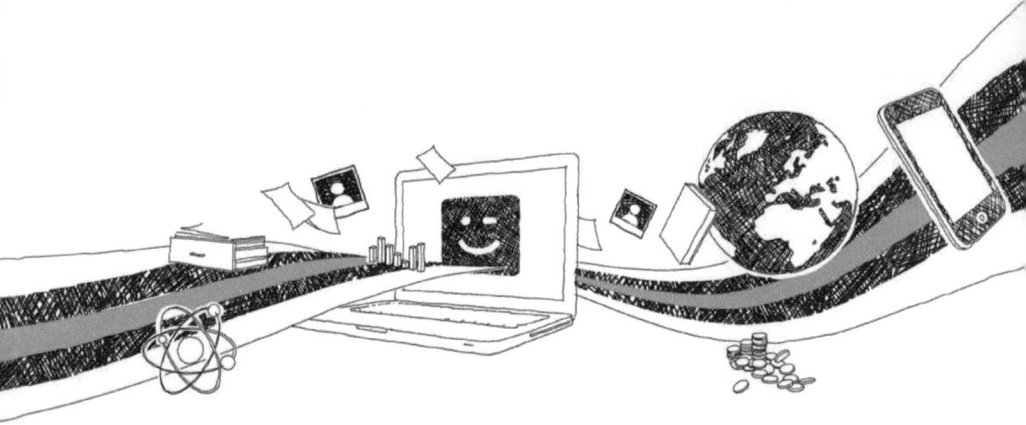
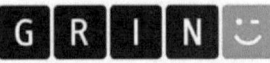